T0131616

48 HOUR FAT BURN SOLUTION

Lose inches of body fat on demand

MILES BECCIA

BALBOA.
PRESS

A DIVISION OF HAY HOUSE

Copyright © 2016 Miles Beccia.

All rights reserved. No part of this book may be used or reproduced by any means, graphic, electronic, or mechanical, including photocopying, recording, taping or by any information storage retrieval system without the written permission of the author except in the case of brief quotations embodied in critical articles and reviews.

Balboa Press books may be ordered through booksellers or by contacting:

Balboa Press
A Division of Hay House
1663 Liberty Drive
Bloomington, IN 47403
www.balboapress.com
1 (877) 407-4847

Because of the dynamic nature of the Internet, any web addresses or links contained in this book may have changed since publication and may no longer be valid. The views expressed in this work are solely those of the author and do not necessarily reflect the views of the publisher, and the publisher hereby disclaims any responsibility for them.

The author of this book does not dispense medical advice or prescribe the use of any technique as a form of treatment for physical, emotional, or medical problems without the advice of a physician, either directly or indirectly. The intent of the author is only to offer information of a general nature to help you in your quest for emotional and spiritual well-being. In the event you use any of the information in this book for yourself, which is your constitutional right, the author and the publisher assume no responsibility for your actions.

Any people depicted in stock imagery provided by Thinkstock are models, and such images are being used for illustrative purposes only.
Certain stock imagery © Thinkstock.

Print information available on the last page.

ISBN: 978-1-5043-6488-1 (sc)
ISBN: 978-1-5043-6490-4 (e)

Library of Congress Control Number: 2016913804

Balboa Press rev. date: 11/09/2016

TABLE OF CONTENTS

Introduction vii

Chapter 1. Your Body Is Amazing 1

Chapter 2. Keeping Your Fitness Forward Focus 7

Chapter 3. My Step By Step 48 Hour Fat Burn
Solution 15

Chapter 4. Why Is Your Metabolism So Out Of
Control 25

Chapter 5. Boost Your Fat Burning Aerobics
With Ease 33

Chapter 6. Monitor Your Weight and Keep It
Where You Want It 37

Chapter 7. Minimize Your Stress for Continued
Weight Loss Success 41

Conclusion - Do It Now, Don't Wait 45

INTRODUCTION

I guarantee that the information I will present to you in this book will help you make an amazing breakthrough in your life. I have found that my clients love this because they can get back to eating some of the same foods their grandparents or great-grandparents ate before canned, processed, and refined food supplies changed the way we shop and put our meals together. Are you ready for a cultural shift?

You body is amazing! Each day your body systems adapt and change to environmental conditions. You can gain weight, lose weight, gain strength, lose strength, improve flexibility, or get tight muscles causing injury. My goal is for you to truly understand the relationship you have with your body. Food intake and physical activity can change your fitness and health for yourself and your family for the rest of your lifes.

When I was a teenager, my frustration was to learn how to regain muscle strength and coordination needed to play sports that I loved once again after it was lost from suffering two broken legs from being struck by an automobile in an intersection. After lying in a hospital bed for over three months, I was released with zero muscle to stand or walk. I remember vividly how I tried to lift either leg off the bed and no matter how much I wanted to neither one would move.

When I got out of the hospital with no muscle function in my lower body, my grandpa had to use a fireman's carry to get me up the steps into the house. I was in a wheelchair and struggled to learn how to stand on my own two feet. The support of my family, friends, and the wonderful physical therapy staff got me back on my feet and after another six months I did not have to use crutches anymore. That was an education in patience. From there, I didn't know just how long it would take to regain my athletic talents.

Following this recovery phase, I failed to perform the as well as I previously had in my favorite sports on the playing field. This was very disappointing. At the time, I had no means to change that, so I resolved to let my favorite sports go until I could figure out how to recovery my physical capacity.

The first big change I noticed was the following summer, as I rode my bike about an hour back and forth to work each day. I also ate better, with breakfast, lunch, and dinner, and I began to build more physical stamina in my muscles. In high school, when my physics teacher described how every bone is a lever and every muscle is a hydraulic piston that holds a position and moves the lever using energy, I realized that I could put the pieces together to make my muscles work to move me where I wanted them to go. In spite of this huge setback, I could still actually achieve my goal of competing as a college athlete!

I started surrounding myself with others who had trained hard and eaten well to build the muscle that I desired to have. Learning how to get into great physical condition was my goal. I really started taking note that the better I ate real whole foods and performed my exercises properly this was propelling me forward as I was shaping my body and mind.

During college, I had started working at fitness centers and learning new exercise programs. I worked through every training program I could find: Olympic weightlifting, powerlifting, martial arts, flag football, rugby, Pilates, yoga, aerobic step classes, swimming, mountain biking, and body building. I met many outstanding athletes and people over those years who are still my friends today.

I majored in Public Health Education and was grateful to be able to participate in college athletics in both track and field and football. My dietary intake at that time required an enormous amount of food to maintain all that physical activity. While in college, I competed as an amateur bodybuilder and powerlifter, so the training for these competitions increased my caloric and food intake needs.

After my success as a competitive college athlete, my life changed and my physical activity slowed down. My struggle with weight control began after college. I began working each day to help others improve their physical capacity and eat better, yet I kept eating the same numbers of large meals I had as an athlete. No surprise, then, when I began to steadily gain more and more body weight. One day I stepped on the scale and was shocked when the readout announced my weight as 248 pounds. I had continued to see myself as a lean, strong adult role model, and this weight did not match my vision.

I knew I needed to change my eating habits.

I knew I didn't want to eat five or six meals a day, because it wasn't healthy for my digestive system to work all day long and it left me hungry all day. When I realized that my former mindset and eating program no longer worked for me, I was determined to learn more about the human body and make certain I could achieve my weight loss goal. I recalled the feelings of failure I had experienced when I didn't make the baseball or golf teams in college: I was miserable. I needed to solve my nutrition planning to help me get back my athletic physical condition.

Now everything I had learned up to this point and getting up to date research would lead me back to the optimal health I had achieved as a collegiate athlete. I found the key to keeping my energy levels up naturally, having enough energy for recuperation, and staying focused was to eat better and better *real* whole foods in specific combinations of dietary fiber. I began with Italian American foods, because that's what I was most familiar with, but soon I started to use new recipes and methods of cooking to bring in excellent nutrition.

I focused on everything I'd learned about the digestive processes when I was studying health education at the university, particularly how our body works to bring in food, break it down to absorb all the nutrition possible, and then eliminate wastes. I began to see that the body is like a manufacturing plant, providing us energy and eliminating the byproducts. Digestion works like any managed process so that it can not be moving too quickly or slowly. That pattern is central to every part of our digestive processes.

Once I realized how much weight I had gained, I did not start performing all the same intense physical activities I had done during my college years. Rather, I focused on portion control for breakfast, lunch, and dinner. At the end of 8 weeks, using the same routine you are reading about right now, I stepped on the scale and it read a steady 217. Yes, that was a 31 pound deficit, and 3.9 pounds per week of weight loss. I did not lose any endurance or strength from my normal activities during this time, and it fit with my future fitness vision for myself, so I have maintained that weight ever since.

Now I want you to think in a new way about how a healthy body weight starts in *your* gut. It starts in your gut because your healthy digestive system runs from your stomach all way through the breakdown of foods, nourishment of your body, and then elimination of wastes. So, you might ask, what does it mean to have a healthy gut?

Your gut is ineffective without dietary fiber. Yet many diet programs focus on protein, fat, or sugar levels. I want you to focus on having a balanced intake of dietary fiber. To create a healthy gut, we need two types of dietary fiber: soluble and insoluble fiber.

Soluble fiber forms a gel in water. This makes all the food that sits in your stomach become a ball (or bolus) of food. Insoluble fiber does not break down during digestion but is there to cleanse and clean the walls of the gut from top to bottom to maintain a healthy environment. The insoluble fiber intake tends to speed up your digestion, while the soluble fiber tends to clump your meal together to moderate the speed of digestion.

This is the basis of my proven weight control program and ultimately how fit you look and feel going forward throughout your lifetime. The next chapter discusses the relationship between soluble and insoluble fiber in detail.

Keep reading and you will begin to understand the most important concepts of my 48 Hour Fat Burn Solution plan in more detail.

Write out what you can image you see of your physical condition in the photos at your 80th birthday party. Describe in vivid detail your posture, skin appearance, muscle tone, etc.

_____

_____

_____

_____

Chapter One

YOUR BODY IS AMAZING

48 hours on a restricted-calorie diet is all your body can withstand before you begin moving into a starvation state. You probably know how this feels because it is the point other fad diets need you to get past in order to really accelerate your weight loss. *AND*, this is the point when most rapid weight loss fad diets fail.

The problem with moving into a starvation phase is that it sets up the body for large amounts of fat storage right after the next big harvest time – that is, when you finally begin eating those yummy full feeling meals again. Yes, remember your body is amazing. It can gain weight, lose weight, lose muscle, gain muscle, and go all directions as we go through life.

After 2 to 3 days of restricting your calorie intake, your body moves into the state of ketosis. Ketosis is the process of creating substances called ketones as the body breaks down fat for energy. Ketosis is a sign that our body has shifted into starvation mode and is beginning to using alternative sources of energy, rather than the standard ones we use when we have a healthy, stable, balanced nutritional intake.

When you haven't taken in enough normal amounts of carbohydrates from food for your cells to burn for energy, your body begins supplying itself with energy instead. The body controls its energy supply in multiple ways, so when you are healthy and eating a balanced diet, you don't make or use ketones. However, when you cut way back on your calories or carbs, your body will switch to ketosis for energy. When your body kicks into this mode, it is slowing down your previously elevated metabolism and is setting you up to store lots of fat once you begin eating normally again.

So why do so many diet programs carry us to the brink of failure with these long, arduous days, weeks, or months where our body is in starvation mode, only to end by storing so much extra fat afterwards? Well, it's because in the short term, restricting calories works – you can get results from changing your calorie intake.

More than likely, you've tried these diets not once, but several times. What you need to realize is that this process is hurting you, and it is never going to give you the lasting results you're seeking. On average, 80 percent to 90 percent of people who use these kinds of calorie-restricting diets regain the weight they lost. Many gain even more back. This is why it's crucial to understand the internal science of how our body responds to restricted calories.

The way to alter this pattern is with choice. The choice to start with a balanced breakfast, lunch, and dinner for the metabolism you are at today. Another problem is that most people fail to monitor whether they're losing, gaining, or staying at the same weight day to day or week to week. Without monitoring your progress, it's hard to know which portion sizes or numbers of calories will help you reach and keep you at the place you want to be.

Case Study:

Maggie is a busy working mom and new grandmother. She knew that her time was limited so that meant she really must set up her daily schedule to accommodate some physical activities and a better meal plan. In her experiences up to now, Maggie had tried just about everything to stay trim and fit for her to be a great example to her kids and family.

She once was a runner and at that point in her life she had more time along with an environment to get out on the road for a run each morning. This gave her more focus toward eating healthy foods to maintain her energy. She came in frustrated with the way she looked and felt. After providing her with the fitness and nutrition stages of progression, she began immediately. Maggie's focus now to move through these stages of success and reclaim her health and fitness from here onward.

She had agreed that just starving herself did not work in the past and she knew that the only way to navigate her way was to do it smart. This empowered Maggie to set time for her physical conditioning of muscle endurance and aerobic improvement along with her following the guidelines set out here in the 48 Hour Fat Burn Solution. Not only did inches of body fat change the shape of her body, but she came in one day so pumped up about how easy it was for her to pick up her kayak compared to the struggle it was prior to her beginning the program with me.

Now, I do have some bad news. The thing is that focusing long and hard on your weight loss is not enough to create the success you seek. We often hear that it takes 21 days to change a habit, but that's really a bit of nonsense.

If you have been on the typical trend of gaining 10 or more pounds per decade since you stopped growing in height, between the ages of 17 and 21, it will take more than 21 days to gain the knowledge and the practice of how to shop, store, prepare, and eat the right portions of real foods to see yourself have lasting success.

The *48 Hour Fat Burn Solution* is a program that will change your eating habits for the rest of your life. This program will improve your total health in measurable ways. As you continue my program, you will see the results at your periodic medical exams, as well as in your daily activities and interests.

Those who do not begin immediately to make changes to their meal plan and physical activity daily will be putting themselves into an environment which is ripe for sickness, disease, and poor state of mind. Each of you who sets up a nutritious meal plan and performs purposeful physical activities will find yourself with an abundance of energy, freedom from lasting illness, and a vibrant state of mind.

Write out what you will see yourself being able to do 6 months from now after you lose body fat and improve your physical fitness. Describe in vivid detail your posture, muscle tone, clothing appearance, etc.

_____

_____

_____

_____

Chapter Two

KEEPING YOUR FITNESS FORWARD FOCUS

The vital combination of factors which must be learned, practiced, and maintained for you to free yourself from a tired, injured, and simply unhealthy body is the culture or growth of fitness and nutrition within you and your environment. Having a kitchen set up for meal preparation, cooking, and storage is a system within itself that will make you happy to be in when things are in the right place or miserable with frustration along with hunger when you do not have each area working properly.

Same holds true for when you have for easy access to physical activities which you can truly look forward to doing on autopilot when designed and practiced right. Let us start by seeing what it takes to have enough energy daily to think, work, and have some left over for a workout.

I want you start by considering how a fit, healthy body weight begins in your gut. This is the most important aspect of my 48 Hour Fat Burn Solution. Why is this so important? As discussed, the body is a manufacturing plant that takes in raw materials, processes them to produce the right energy units (fat or sugar) or building blocks (proteins or amino acids), and eliminates the byproducts.

Your gut is ineffective without both types of dietary fiber. Again, unlike most diets or nutrition plans, we will not be focusing on protein, fat, or sugar intake. Your goal here is to make sure that you have a balanced intake of dietary fiber. To create a healthy gut you need both soluble and insoluble fiber.

These two types of dietary fiber have different roles in maintaining the proper function of your digestive organs. As we touched on earlier, soluble fiber forms gel in the stomach after it is chewed to break it apart. This turns all the food that sits in your stomach into a ball of nutrients that can be used by the body. Insoluble fiber does not break down during digestion; its job is to cleanse the walls of the gut from top to bottom to maintain a healthy environment.

During my early stages of learning how to rebuild my physical conditioning and play sports again, I studied diet and meal plan of every strength athlete I could find. These nutrition plans included olympic weightlifting programs, powerlifting athletes, bodybuilding books, and even Sumo wrestlers because

I needed to gain muscle and body weight. The common equation with all of these sports conditioning plans was to eat a base of healthy foods but in portion sizes large enough to add up to more than I was using for activities each day.

As you can understand this strategy works for them and it worked for me. I steadily gained body weight and kept my energy levels up to perform added physical conditioning programs. One of the most impressive parts of learning these weight gain systems was to see how the bodybuilder worked the strategy to maintain level blood sugar by eating very often and keeping calories very balanced when slowly trimming off body fat. This was the opposite of the Sumo wrestler whose strategy was to skip meals, especially breakfast, to trick the body into low blood sugars to add additional body fat when eating more calories than they used each day.

I used both of these strategies when it came to a season of football which required a higher body weight versus a season of track and field which it was best to have a lower body fat for better speed. From these years of experience and the research I did while studying for my degree in Public Health, I gained an expansive knowledge of how to make changes in both nutrition planning and physical conditioning. Some of the most important pieces came from learning about the history of meal plans from other cultures at all corners of the globe and the past and continuing research with regard to dietary fiber food categories.

The intake of proper soluble dietary fiber is the demonstrated by scientific evidence as the secret to maintaining even blood sugar levels, reducing cholesterol levels, and developing a clean healthy gut. Without properly balanced dietary fiber, you will have improper passage of food, either moving too fast or too slow. This balance of dietary fiber is necessary to maintain a healthy level of digestive bacteria and for overall good health.

You can start now to understand how the passage of food from the stomach to the small intestine for its long track of breakdown and absorption, then into the large intestine for final removal of broken down nutrients, and ultimate passage to the colon is a steady manufacturing process that requires proper setup with the right amounts and types of dietary fiber.

The world has changed rapidly in the past half-century to the point where, on demand, we can now consume giant amounts of calories in just a few minutes, yet hardly any of it contains dietary fiber from healthy foods. The average American diet contains less than one-third of the daily requirement for healthy dietary fiber intake.

In more than 100 countries around the globe, people now follow the pattern of eating too many calories with limited amounts of dietary fiber. These high-calorie, low-fiber foods leave you hungry all the time and create low blood sugar, so almost as soon as you've eaten, you have to run out and get some more to boost you back up. Can you see the problem with this cycle?

A little over a century ago, every individual, family, community, neighborhood, and city would eat food from the fresh local markets that had the dietary fiber needed for a healthy gut. This habit of consuming lower calorie, higher fiber foods is still maintained as a regular meal pattern by many rural families around the globe. These families are in great physical shape, yet their cousins who live in communities that rely on fast food or quick-prep foods suffer with health problems. Poor food patterns and lack of physical activity lead to short- and long-term health problems.

Dietary fiber still shows up in the news on a weekly basis, as it has been an easily available key component of the human diet for thousands of years. Spices, an easily traced dietary component, were one of the first globally traded regular food items. Throughout history, the crops harvested for food supply season by season, and decade after decade, could also be easily traced through cultural migrations and the spice trade.

Spices traveled from East to West and West to East, as flavors followed the water seasons that produced the food supply. We can trace these cultural origins of our food patterns to understand the development of healthy diets. Families in these diverse cultures began to thrive and develop the centers of civilization that gave rise to the healthiest and most successful nations.

These amazing changes happened over a long period in history. We are now seeing a renaissance of healthy eating in the abundance of fresh fruits, vegetables, grains, nuts and seeds, beans and legumes popping up everywhere in local markets. This new model will make it easy to replace the unhealthy processed foods that are have become so readily available. The fact is that every day we have more locally grown and fresh food farms all around us, and we can harvest the best fiber foods from these local markets.

Great things are happening now with grocery stores, restaurants, and even ready-to-go packaged foods offering low calorie portions that contain plenty of dietary fiber. One problem we have, however, is determining which foods and which dietary fibers are going to help us manage our digestion and make us feel full so that we do not feel hungry all the time.

I will help solve that question for you as you read through my Step-by-Step System in the next chapter. There, you will learn my soluble/insoluble fiber solution. The program will indicate the minimum amount of soluble fiber you need to form a gel in your stomach that will manage the time-release nature of your food as it moves through the stomach, small intestine, large intestine, and is ultimately eliminated in a normal pattern of digestion.

I will coach you through your personal food culture shift. Understand that you will likely experience some awkward emotional changes as you gain knowledge through practice and build yourself an easy-to-maintain menu plan of delicious meals you and your family will love. We will do this together.

My easy to follow my step-by-step soluble/insoluble fiber system will take you through a progressive increase in the right amount of dietary fiber to digest the "Beccia Ball" for time-released energy. You will be able to steadily improve your physical capacity for activity and, more importantly, see your waist-to-hip ratio become what you always dreamed it could be.

The abundance of today's food supply for easy, quick, flavorful meals will be the key to sustaining your weight, looking amazing, and having lots of energy to gain greater success throughout your life.

As you put this easy system into practice, you will gain the edge that will give you a tremendous victory in your weight-control battle. Some of you will lose weight easily on my program. Others will continue to seek the full benefits of my program that will help you transform your digestive process so that you can see the visible results in your health. I know you're still here with me because you're no longer looking for the quick fix. You want concrete information, principles, and techniques that will ensure you are on the right success track to reach your destination.

Write out below what you already make for a meal which is in you family cultural history prior to modern refrigeration. (If you are not sure, please ask someone near you about their experience.)

_____

_____

_____

_____

Chapter Three

MY STEP BY STEP 48 HOUR FAT BURN SOLUTION

I will now coach you through my step-by-step system. Learning to focus on the single task of burning body fat in short intervals and monitoring your weight in between the fat-burn intervals will ensure success in shifting your personal metabolism. I will walk you through how the science of natural energy manufacture and waste elimination applies to you to ensure that your digestion follows a continuous, consistent path for lasting success.

My proven system of 48 Hour Fat Burn intervals, during which you consume nutritious high-fiber foods that are abundant and easily available to you, has benefited my clients and will be your key to a vibrant new you.

I previously introduced the concept that your digestive system needs to be fit and functioning at top efficiency from top to bottom so that every last drop of nutrition will fertilize each and every cell within your body. Additionally, all the waste products from every system in your body – like those that engineer rejuvenation and energy production – must be removed for everything to continue working optimally.

We discussed the fact that optimal health is only possible when your digestive muscle tone is adequate, allowing a consistent digestive transit time (approximately 48 hours) for each meal digestion, which allows the complete processes of food absorption and elimination to occur.

When industrialized nations began moving away from basic daily recipes made with local foods that contained items in the 5 Super Fiber Food Categories (i.e., vegetables, nuts and seeds, fruits, grains, beans and legumes), people started replacing these common-sense meals with high-calorie packaged and canned foods, oversized sandwiches, and enormous sugary drinks. The result from eating like that? Your gut grows slack and leaves you constantly hungry from poor digestion and poor nutrition.

My Soluble Fiber Threshold system sets up enough of a soluble fiber gel to ball up your entire meal into a time release capsule that suppresses your appetite for hours, and throughout the remainder of your day. Starting with your breakfast and at lunch, you must create a ball (or bolus) of food that forms in your stomach and remains there for pre-digestion for anywhere from 1 to 4 hours. The ball of food eventually moves down into your small intestine for actual breakdown through digestion. I call this time-released bolus of pre-digestion soluble fiber in the stomach the "Beccia Ball."

Dietary fiber is extremely important for you to achieve optimal health within your digestive system, yet the average American adult takes in about one-third of the daily requirements. A small portion of fiber is metabolized in the stomach and intestines, while the rest is passed through the intestinal tract and eventually makes up part of the stool. It is necessary to keep your body from becoming overburdened from poor performance in both the areas of nutrient absorption and waste removal. This is usually seen when bowel transit time is either too slow or too fast.

I already described the two types of dietary fiber: soluble fiber and insoluble fiber. The current recommendation is to eat between 25 and 35 grams (g) of total fiber each day. The thing is, until now no distinction has been made between the two types, nor reference any to the need to balance the two. Yet it is being proven that the balance of soluble and insoluble fiber is the key to achieving optimal health at any age.

Remember how I described how soluble fiber combines with water and turns to gel during digestion. This slows digestion and food absorption in the stomach and intestine, which creates a timed release of sugar into the blood that helps keep blood sugars down. This gel also binds with cholesterol during digestion and removes it from the bloodstream.

Your 3 Step Daily Plan to Unlock Secret 48 Hour Fat Burn Recipe

1. Suppress your appetite by making a "Beccia Ball" time-released Soluble Fiber Threshold capsule made of real soluble fiber solution foods from my 5 Super Fiber Food Categories for breakfast and lunch. Then eat your regular dinner!
2. During the 48 hours, eat 3 meals per day that total approximately 65 percent of the daily recommended calorie intake for active adults. [Eat a total of 1,430 calories/day for women; 1,855 calories/day for men.]
3. Hydrate your digestive system by drinking 16 to 24 ounces of water between meals.

5 Super Fiber Food Categories

1. Vegetables
2. Nuts and seeds
3. Fruits
4. Beans and legumes
5. Grains

I'll show you how you'll use combinations of these 5 Super Fiber Food Categories to suppress your appetite, eat fewer calories by using spices and seasonings, and create a healthy gut which will help you control your weight.

My step-by-step program will teach you to monitor your fat loss during 48 hour intervals, while eating delicious foods that are a natural appetite suppressant and which enable you to burn fat as your main fuel source.

The *48 Hour Fat Burn Solution* employs my original discovery of the Soluble Fiber Threshold for properly form a "Beccia Ball" in your stomach. You need a minimum of 4 grams of soluble fiber from 3 of the 5 Super Fiber Food Categories. This will enable your body signals to readjust as you create a healthy digestive pattern that essentially restores you to proper digestive continuity.

The calendar you see below is an example of how to make steady step by step successful drops in body fat while you can eat anything you want as long as you are monitoring you body weight like I will be describing in more detail in a later chapter. Your body knows when you are low in blood sugar for too long and that is why this strategy will trick it from the rapid fat building of a starvation diet.

48-Hour Fat Burn Monthly Calendar

Sunday	Monday	Tuesday	Wednesday	Thursday	Friday	Saturday
1 OFF	2 REDUCE	3 REDUCE	4 OFF	5 REDUCE	6 REDUCE	7 OFF
8 OFF	9 REDUCE	10 REDUCE	11 OFF	12 REDUCE	13 REDUCE	14 OFF
15 OFF	16 REDUCE	17 REDUCE	18 OFF	19 REDUCE	20 REDUCE	21 OFF
22 OFF	23 REDUCE	24 REDUCE	25 OFF	26 REDUCE	27 REDUCE	28 OFF

The most important benefit of soluble fiber from each food group is that it creates this bolus of food, the "Beccia Ball," that keeps you feeling full longer and encourages the smooth muscles of your digestive tract to perform peristalsis (smooth muscle cell contractions) to move this ball through your system. This results in the use of additional energy for digesting your food as your smooth muscles are forced to adapt and get in shape (i.e., increased resting metabolism).

Soluble fiber is found in foods that are less common in our daily menu choices. The new foods you will enjoy daily include oatmeal, oat bran, barley, oranges, grapefruit, pears, nuts, flax seeds, sunflower seeds, beans, peas, blueberries, raisins, grapes, other fruits, psyllium, zucchini, celery, broccoli, cabbage, onions, and carrots.

The job of insoluble fiber is to speed up the passage of foods through the stomach and intestines and add bulk to the stool. In general, this can be very irritating to your digestive system and keep you always feeling hungry. This type of fiber is found in many of our daily menu choices. Going forward, you will now combine the consumption of foods like whole wheat, wheat bran, lentils, seeds, nuts, couscous, tomatoes, dark leafy vegetables, and root vegetable skins with higher soluble fiber foods.

As success begins to motivate you, the time will come for you to test your progress and creativity. Look at replacing just one or all the items to create a meal with balanced fiber that you will enjoy eating with those around you. View each meal prep as if you were making it to serve to others or ordering it when eating out.

Success Steps

– Step 1 –

Begin each meal with your soluble fiber foods that will create a layer of food "Beccia Ball" for a timed release of energy and appetite suppression between meals.

– Step 2 –

Measure and record your portions enough times so that you understand what the correct amount is for you to first lose body fat, and then maintain your weight loss.

– Step 3 –

Plan ahead. Planning your food consumption for the day is absolutely crucial to successfully using the 48-Hour Fat Burn Solution. It will help eliminate the frustration of knowing what you **should** be eating when your supply is not readily available. If you know you will be on the go, be proactive and set up a travel bag with the correct portions of food for each meal.

Day 1 – Breakfast & Lunch

Breakfast Female (1430 cal.) & Male (1855 cal.)	Lunch Female (1430 cal.)	Lunch Male (1855 cal.)
1 ounce almonds, no salt (22 almonds) 1 cup carrots 1 cup strawberries, raw ½ medium banana, raw	¾ cup brown rice, cooked (no salt or fat added) 1½ cups cooked broccoli ½ cup kidney beans, canned (no fat added) 1 cup grapes	1 cup brown rice, cooked (no salt or fat added) 2 cups cooked broccoli ¾ cup kidney beans, canned (no fat added) 1 cup grapes
Dinner – Female (1430 cal.) & Male (1855 cal.)		
Eat your regular, sensible dinner		

Day 2 – Breakfast & Lunch

Breakfast Female (1430 cal.) & Male (1855 cal.)	Lunch Female (1430 cal.)	Lunch Male (1855 cal.)
1 medium orange, raw) 1 ounce walnuts (14 halves) 1 cup carrots	¾ medium potato, cooked, (no salt or fat added) 1 cup sliced carrots 2 cups green beans ¼ ounce almonds (dry roasted, no salt) ½ medium grapefruit	1 medium potato, cooked, (no salt or fat added) 1 cup sliced carrots 2 cups green beans ½ ounce almonds (dry roasted, no salt) ½ medium grapefruit
Dinner – Female (1430 cal.) & Male (1855 cal.)		
Eat your regular, sensible dinner		

Write out one fresh dietary fiber whole food that you would love to have on your plate for breakfast, lunch, and dinner today. (Make note to where you can purchase these foods in a ready to eat package.)

_____

_____

_____

_____

Chapter Four

WHY IS YOUR METABOLISM SO OUT OF CONTROL

Your appetite is keeping you overweight. The biggest key to success on the *48 Hour Fat Burn Solution* is learning your best portion size to maintain a steady body weight in between your intervals. As I mentioned in the Introduction, exercise is not the most important route to weight loss but it essential because your muscles are your biggest metabolizers or users of energy.

Physical activities are required for balancing your energy stores within your muscle and fat cells, as well as maintaining your best body metabolism which I will describe in more detail here. The daily calorie requirements I have set up in this plan have been put together using the lifelong sum of an active female and an active male.

You portion size and dietary intake are the key factors to lasting weight control. I will coach you toward the proper portions for your body and train you to achieve the proper balance for optimal muscle and aerobic capacity. As a result, you will feel better and be happy with your weight control and energy level.

Why can I eat so much at one time and not even be hungry?

Our primitive human harvest season mindset and actual biology says to eat as much as you can until the big harvest is gone. If harvest lasted one month anytime prior to modern storage systems, then you would eat and eat until you add on ten or more pounds because it could be six months before the food supply is back. Most everyone was told to keep eating until your plate is empty! Even though the reality is that most of us are in a constant state of harvest with no end in sight.

We will now focus foremost on the engineering, which is by far the only way to make the digestive system come together and efficiently reward you with the results you are seeking. As you practice eating the correct portions of food with the right weekly total calorie intake, you will feel lasting freedom from the immense stress of fighting the battle of a bulging waistline.

Your goal is to take in 65 percent of your total calories expended for the day during the *48 Hour Fat Burn Interval*. Your body will burn away stored fat for the remaining

35 percent of energy supply during this phase of partial calorie restriction. Your calories will be split among a daily eating pattern of 3 main meals and a snack, if needed, to provide your body the food necessary for your fat release mechanism to achieve full release mode. This pattern allows your digestive organs a longer rest period between meals to rest and destress from using energy.

This is a natural law or principle that is as reliable as is gravity. When you apply it properly to alter your "lifestyle" planning and set yourself up for a new culture, this will make all other practical tools more powerful and more useful. It will also make your goal attainment easier, more certain, and more permanent.

Your Resting Metabolic Rate (RMR) is actually not a fixed number of calories. The energy needs of your body and mind are constantly shifts up and down, depending upon multiple factors, such as total lean body mass, daily physical activity, hydration, blood glucose levels, stress level, and many additional issues. Your lasting success is derived by managing your weight control after determining your personal shifts in your which is now been slightly renamed your Thermodynamic Metabolic Rate.

The range of calories required for you to lose, maintain, or gain body fat and body weight is constantly shifting up and down. You need to measure and understand the portions of food you are eating to make sure your personal calorie level is on target to either lose, maintain, or gain body fat.

Now think back to when you were keeping a closer watch with your portions and how active your where. I truth as you can see throughout this book is that a female has less muscle mass, due to lack of testosterone, than a male does. A women has to be closer on target with portion control and physical activities to make her calorie burning rate stay elevated. A male who stays somewhat close to portion size and does just enough physical activity to tap into his muscle mass from testosterone get to melt away the body fat.

Remember your body is amazing, so now matter what condition you are in now it is a guarantee of mine that by combining the fitness and nutrition systems I am outlining here you will see and feel exponential benefits in your health. You must continue to read the rest of the chapters to learn the special aerobic endurance techniques that sets this plan apart from others you have done or seen before.

Any successful project begins by following the footsteps of those who have already been able to achieve your desired result. If you do not make a menu that utilizes your favorite flavor combinations, you will quickly revert back to bad foods that will cause you gain back any weight you have put such hard work into losing.

Working on mastering the meals provided in the correct portions and cooking your food the way you like it and flavored as if you were eating at your favorite restaurant is not rocket science. I will help you use low-calorie, no-salt seasonings from your favorite cuisines – Italian, Mexican, Thai, Greek, and any others you like. You'll start by setting up your pantry and seasoning cabinet, which will get you off on the right foot toward success.

In the beginning, my favorite flavors were Italian American because those were what I experienced growing up in my family. You will bring your favorite family recipes to this program.

Today we have access to thousands of recipes reflecting every cultural diversity in every nation around the globe. What are some of your favorites? How can you integrate those flavors and recipes into your regular healthy meals? Employing your favorite flavors is the key to success and will enable you to enjoy tasty, healthy meals that keep you on this eating program.

As you learn and use these methods and strategies, you will avoid the anxiety of having to suffer through yet another distasteful diet. My eating program will actually taste great. Better still, as you see your tummy flatten, you will not have to count every calorie or point to look and feel great while you maintain your weight loss and eat REAL foods that are flavored just the way you like them.

How does water help your fat burning process? The internal manufacturing plant that is your digestive system can shut down from a lack of water. The lack of water acts paradoxically as a dampening agent and, in effect, extinguishes your fat burning for energy. Your body must have the water it needs to support healthy digestion for the fat-burning flames to blaze at their hottest for the full 48 hours.

Let's explore how this applies directly to you. In general, your muscles maintain your metabolism. When you experience even slight dehydration of just a few ounces of water, your metabolism and performance are reduced. Water is the medium through which chemical reactions take place, and it will either limit or support your body's ability to process nutrition in your gut, burn away fat in your muscles, and remove waste.

During digestion, you must also practice maintaining low levels of any type of stress until the effective breakdown of your food is accomplished.

One major change with regard to water is learning to drink a minimum of 16 to 24 ounces of water (yes, low or no-calorie flavored water is great) at least 60 to 90 minutes before each meal to hydrate your digestive tract. This will set up the best environment to process or "hack" food breakdown and eliminate wastes from not just the digestive tract, but from all body systems. Always have a full bottle of water with you!

The next most important step is to drink small mouthfuls of water during your meal to set up the layer of soluble fiber in your stomach. After the meal is done, you will simply let this layer sit as long as needed to move naturally into small intestine.

The best advice for staying hydrated properly is learn to observe a state of dehydration, which is indicated by your urine color. As you read this, you already know you are a different size and shape from everyone around you, so how can there be a standard of "just drink one gallon a day" for everyone? There is no such one-size-fits-all standard. You must simply look at your urine in the morning and the afternoon to see what color it is. Ideally, if you are well hydrated, your urine will be very light yellow to clear.

If you do are unable to produce any urine to observe, you are already dehydrated and must start drinking water until you have some urine output to observe. Each time you go to the restroom, simply take a look. When the color is too dark, start to drink more water so that the next time it is lighter in color. When you observe a normal light color, you can slow down and consume normal amounts of water that satisfy your thirst.

Write out below one or two practical methods of portions control that you have already used during a weight management program.

_____

_____

_____

_____

Chapter Five

BOOST YOUR FAT BURNING AEROBICS WITH EASE

Normally you would consider the harder your body works at burning calories during moderate to intense physical activities, the better off you would be for fat burning. The key to looking like a conditioned triathlete or a marathon runner is to slowly improve your fitness capacity but with a slower heart rate and comfortable breath rate. So a higher output for longer with a lower overall exertion level is the key to fat burning for energy instead of burn out of sugar and being tired all the time.

Your muscle energy or metabolism from physical activities comes from fat and sugar. Each muscle cell has some energy converters or what is called a mitochondria which takes fat and sugar and turns it into energy to flex your muscle cell. Unfortunately, you do have to train your body to use fat as the most efficient and effective energy source. But as I have said your body is amazing and you can do this so don't wait.

Since fat has more calories, at 9 calories per gram versus 4 calories per gram for sugar, your body is happier when it is energized with more than DOUBLE the energy supply. As you get stronger and improve your (1) gas exchange or lung capacity, (2) heart volume from strength and endurance of cardiac muscle, and (3) blood circulation of the muscles out and back to your heart, you will notice your heart rate becoming lower at the same intensity of exercise. This is called your VO2, or volume of oxygen consumed, and indicates that you are increasing the amount of fat burned during physical activity.

Use the details of the following muscle endurance aerobic fat burn plan to remove the anxiety and hesitation about aerobic activities and use my Breathing O2 Flow Pattern to feed the flames of the fat burning inside your muscles. Your muscles will burn fat for energy only when oxygen is available. Hence the term *aerobic*, which means that oxygen paired with fatty acids combines to burn energy. Failing to improve and maintain your physical activity will lead to another struggle with keeping your body fat at a healthy level.

I would like to have you begin with conditioning how to breath like an endurance swimmer, runner, or bicycle pro. This is also very similar to the method in which yoga breath work is taught as well because some yoga classes are very fast moving and become a very tough workout when performed properly with a full breath.

The objective is to pull in a full volume of fresh oxygen smoothly to the bottom of your lungs, where the largest area of the lungs are surrounding your heart, and feel for a slight moment that you have compressed the air in. It is preferred that you bring in the air through the nose on a 3 second pull in and then release the air out on a 3 second count out. This is a 6 second smooth breath that requires muscles to work around your rib cage and in your diaphragm muscle under the lungs.

This O2 Flow breath allows for a more complete oxygen saturation of your blood and sets you up for 10 breaths per minute. I teach everyone to focus on this for the first 10 minutes of aerobic workouts or 100 breaths to set your muscles up for the best chance to burn an elevated level of fat instead of relying on sugar use for energy.

In the process of getting any workout movement going you need to be listening to how your muscles are feeling with proper posture and muscle pattern. This process of improvement in muscle movement pattern is what I call the mind muscle memory system. When you sense a proper flexing and stretching of your target muscles you must memorize the feel and control during that workout session and future physical activity. The saying perfect practice makes perfect has some application here, but if you don't use it you will lose it is the sad reality.

Lifelong activities include but not limited to swimming, walking, hiking, jogging, bicycling, rowing, dancing, and other aerobic conditioning physical activities. Get started now, don't wait.

– Step 1 –

Begin walking, biking, or using an elliptical machine at a slow to medium pattern.

– Step 2 –

Focus on using your lungs at full capacity with each breath by concentrating on the flexibility of the front and back of your rib cage.

– Step 3 –

Perform this activity at least one or two times a day for 100 breaths to fan the flames of your muscle aerobic fat burn.

Write out one physical activity that you can do inside you home and one that you have always enjoyed outside.

_____

_____

_____

_____

Chapter Six

MONITOR YOUR WEIGHT AND KEEP IT WHERE YOU WANT IT

Once you begin to see success shedding pounds, it's important to continue the trend. You can maintain total control of your fat loss and body weight by consistently monitoring your weight change while you are on my *48 Hour Fat Burn Solution*. This will ensure that you maintain a high metabolism and that you do revert to fat storage.

The most important tool for success on this program of body fat loss, weight loss, fat reduction, etc. is an accurate scale to measure your body weight. The change in measurement of your waist and hips is also directly correlated to your desired loss of stored body fat. As you begin the *48 Hour Fat Burn Solution*, you will need a working knowledge of your body weight so that you have a good understanding of when to take action in the event of future weight gain.

Your personal record of your weight and a comparison of body measurements will show you what you need to do to manage your weight gain and/or loss. You can use the monthly calendar chart provided in the earlier chapter to monitor your weight loss on the morning after two days of calorie reduction.

The more accurate records you keep of your body weight as your body fat decreases due to your diet and workout formula, the higher your probability for success. Keeping consistent records is the easiest method for evaluating your continued success because it will alert you to the need to take steps to reverse even a slight weight gain.

Things to keep in mind when choosing a scale:

- **Small, incremental measurements**. Scales with smaller increments offer more accurate readings. The better scales use increments of 0.2 pounds.
- **Multi-user memory capacity**. If you will be sharing the scale with another family member, you may want to purchase a scale that has an internal or cloud-based memory, which can store historical data for more than one user.
- **Large, backlit display**. It can be difficult to read the display on a scale that sits at your feet. Better bathroom scales offer larger displays with backlighting, which are easier to read in dim lighting.

You will get the most reliable results if you take your measurements under consistent conditions: for example, the last thing before you go to bed, always in your underwear, or first thing in the morning as you're ready to step into the shower. Constantly moving a scale can make for inaccurate measurements. A digital scale will work best if you keep it in the same place for all measurements, so chose a spot that's easy to reach but which won't cause a tripping hazard.

Your weight will always have some daily shifts, due to water hydration, amount of food consumed, and waste eliminated. This should not be a surprise or shock you because you will already understand your trend from monitoring your weight changes. Developing this practical understanding of when you need to re-establish a calorie deficit and/or begin additional aerobic workouts will help keep you on course for weight loss success.

If you see a few pounds above your normal 3- to 6-pound variance, you'll know to immediately return to the "65 Percent Menu Plan" and increased aerobic workouts to reverse the weight gain. When you have burned off that extra body fat, resume eating your active calorie level to maintain a zero net weight gain for each week, month, and years to come.

Some important things to remember:

- Do not expect to be perfect in all areas every day while you're on this program.

- Predetermine a solution for the times you move off course before it happens, because it inevitably will.
- Develop and utilize your willpower to act assertively, confidently knowing each action you need to take.
- Practice relaxing before you eat, work out, and especially prior to sleep.

Write out how much your body weight is at this moment and then begin recording what is happening each day. (Make note to how you feel and respond to positive and negative changes.)

_____

_____

_____

_____

Chapter Seven

MINIMIZE YOUR STRESS FOR CONTINUED WEIGHT LOSS SUCCESS

The objective of this program is not to reach a specific weight goal, so please **do not** set one. Your goal is to find out what is possible for you to accomplish when all of your body systems are funneled toward removing stored body fat. When you follow this itinerary properly, your body will begin releasing stored fat energy and you will have success in this challenge – and also for the rest of your life. My *48 Hour Fat Burn Solution* removes stored fat as you preserve and energize lean muscle, which is where you hold the majority of your stored water, as well.

You will have become successful with portioning your food when you can remove 1-3 pounds of body weight in a full 48 hours. You will have become successful with your weight control when you can keep your body weight even on the scale for more than 8 weeks.

When you have completed the *48 Hour Fat Burn Solution* and have taken your final measurements, it will be time to determine a goal for no more than 28 days. After you see what your results are, you can set a reasonable goal for yourself and do the math. You will see what is possible from looking over your itinerary and final results. Only then can you be certain that the goal you outline is one that will make you feel emotionally successful for the next month, next year, and 10 years from now.

Stress sets up the fight-or-flight responses and makes it difficult to follow through with a new eating plan. When you experience some of life's inevitable stress, you will have a choice to get out of the stress the easy way with a quick fix, or staying the course on your new healthy eating plan. Going back to comfort foods is the easy way to relieve stress. Staying with your new eating plan may be difficult until it becomes routine or habit, but it will give you the best long-term results.

Any time you feel your emotions beginning to rise to a stress tipping point, look down at your hands or in the mirror to self-reflect. Are you clenching or tightening your hands? This is a stress to muscle physical response and is nothing more than your signal to reflect. Reflect on what may be causing this stress response and then work to RE-CONstruct your response. You've got two options: (1) the easy way out or (2) the more difficult way of continuing your healthy eating practice until improvement happens. You do not have to be perfect in your head or on paper to know which is the healthier, better decision.

Sometimes life is hard. But you've already experienced many successes in your past, or you wouldn't be here today. I know you have what it takes to stand up to life's new stresses with the courage that has worked for you in your past successes in other key areas of your life. The nutrition plan I am presenting to you in this manual is yours to keep forever and pass down as a way of building lasting fitness and health for you and for your family.

Don't let another day or another excuse go by. Start now!

Success Tools You Will Need

- Monthly supplies of your favorite cuisine flavors
- Seasonings such as cinnamon, honey, vinegar, Italian herbs, capers, mustard, chili powder, tabasco, and red pepper
- A scale for measuring each portion of uncooked and cooked food
- Storage containers for all cooked food or pre-prepped ingredients
- A daily supply of water in your favorite no-calorie flavors (e.g., tea, coffee, lemon, lime, cranberry)

CONCLUSION - DO IT NOW, DON'T WAIT

Now that you know what to do to achieve success, you will find that you fit into this system because it works for you.

My step-by-step system will focus you on the single task of burning off body fat in short intervals and monitoring your weight in between the intervals to ensure your success with today's metabolism. My proven system of 48 Hour Fat Burn intervals during which you eat nutritious high-fiber foods that are abundant everywhere you go is your key to a vibrant new you.

Start this plan NOW and you will see results immediately! As you go through the program, you will learn what the stress signal of discomfort in your tummy actually means. During this plan, the pain in your tummy will raise the question as to whether you should leave the food alone in your stomach to preset a healthy digestion pattern or it's telling you "I'm hungry." You will teach your body that even when you feel hunger, YOU DO NOT have to stuff yourself.

With this program, you will find you have plenty of energy to focus on lasting success with portion control intervals.

It's time to waken your metabolism! Your body does not slow down as you get older, yet your metabolism speeds up and slows down on a daily and hourly basis. This so-called "new" term for this is thermodynamic metabolism.. It means that depending on multiple factors, your body will use more or less energy throughout each day. Today your body may register using 1,753 calories while yesterday, with more sleep and less activity, it would have registered using only 1,604.

When food is more abundant, sleep is good, you have a lower stress response, and you increase your physical activity a bit, your body shifts up a few gears. This means when you restrict your intake of nutritious food for even just a few extra days past my recommended 48 hours – and certainly any longer than a week – or sit around without doing any extra activity, you will feel tired all day and your body will amazingly shift into slow gear.

You now have the know-how and tools so that even when you choose to eat out a few times a week, you have the insight and understanding to choose the best foods to maintain excellent health. Now for the reality part: you must continuously work to stay physically active, and these are the only foods that will support your improved physical activity levels throughout your life.

Following the steps in this program will help you to change your body in ways you would never believe! This is the exact program I used with great success in my own journey to a fit and healthy body. As soon as you get started, you will see why my clients have been using my methods since the early 1990's with lasting success. Most of us need some coaching to break out of the ruts we have been stuck in for years. Through this book, I am now your coach.

As you read this, I know that your past experiences, some bad and some good, may come flooding back to you and cause emotions to rise up. Understand that is OK. It is normal to experience emotions that may cause you to consider not following through with all my steps and techniques. You've tried dieting before and it just didn't work. What's going to be different here?

What's different here is that I have created this system by putting together a number of small success steps. When you perform them consistently, you will have no problem keeping yourself healthy and strong for the rest of your years. You will become even more motivated as action builds momentum and this helps you acquire an enormous mental edge.

Once you reach your weight and fitness goals, you'll know what to do to maintain them. If, at some point, your body is in trouble and your stomach sags, you must again prop yourself up with the routine I have outlined here, and you will soon be looking with excitement for a high five or a fist bump.

Remember to first determine and then focus on the total calories you can take in at what activity level without gaining any body fat, compared to the 48-hour reduced-calorie level of 65 percent. This is now your approximate calorie range to consistently keep the fat off and your fitness up as you continue to monitor yourself. Female calorie intake typically ranges from 1,430 to 2,200, while male calorie intake ranges from 1,855 to 2,900.

The Soluble Fiber Threshold menu plan for this program meets the daily USDA requirements of proteins, fats, and carbohydrates and should become the standard of what you eat each day, even when not trying to remove stored body fat. Now you can add menu food items that are good for you and you enjoy, just as long as you DO NOT start taking in more calories than you expend each day.

Start by following my Soluble Fiber Threshold (SFT), which teaches you to take in 4 grams of soluble fiber at every meal or snack by combining a minimum of 3 different food categories from the 5 Super Fiber Food Categories. As we have established, research shows that soluble fiber creates a timed release ball of food, The Beccia Ball, for better digestion and to help suppress your appetite.

Any change in body weight or inches is a success, and your lasting success is attained by keeping it there. You can now use this new information as your marker in setting realistic goals after completing your best 48 Hour Fat Burn Interval Solution.

Here's to your short-term – and lasting – success!

Printed in the United States
By Bookmasters